My Loved One Has Dementia.

Now What?

Beth Dow

Dedication

To all the caregivers going through this journey now; the caregivers who have not yet begun their journey; and to the caregivers who have completed their journey. In each of you there is endless knowledge, courage, and strength.

In Recognition

I have been blessed with parents, grandparents,
and in-laws who loved me. A husband who
patiently supports me. Sons, daughters-in-law, and
grandchildren who make me so very proud. And
friends, who make life fun.

Table of Contents

Introduction

I am the granddaughter of a woman with vascular dementia. The daughter-in-law of a man who had frontal temporal dementia. The daughter of a woman with Alzheimer's disease. I am the close friend to daughters and sons whose parents have been riddled with one of the many diseases on the dementia spectrum and I have watched them struggle. Through my home care agency, I have seen how the entire family is affected by dementia, not just the one with the diagnosis. Through facilitating support groups, I have seen the toll caregiving takes on the caregiver. Through my teaching, workshops, and seminars, I have seen that even professionals don't know how to best take care of someone with dementia. Through my never-ending thirst for knowledge and to find out everything I can about the person with the disease and those who take care of them, I have found out that, for now, the best weapon we have is knowledge and understanding. And through looking in the eyes of those with dementia, I have learned that the best we can give them are the gifts of respect, patience, love, and understanding that the best way to help them is to go into their world.

My Journey

William D. Pruitt left his family to marry Lucille Parker in 1938. His family told him they would disown him if he married "that woman." *That woman* had a child out of wedlock. In 1938, that was a huge disgrace. He married her anyway. Out of love. He adopted that child and raised her as his own. That child was my mother.

My granddaddy was my hero. A big man. I never doubted his love for me. He used to tell me that when I was born I was the prettiest baby girl in the nursery. He would then smile and say, "Now, you were also the *only* girl in the nursery, but you were still the prettiest." To this day, I have never been more sure of anyone's unconditional love for me than I am of my granddaddy's. Granddaddy loved bigger than any person I have ever known.

Fast forward sixty years. My granddaddy was taking care of my grandmother who, due to a stroke, had vascular dementia. Oh, how he still loved that woman! Granddaddy and Grandmomma lived about an hour and half from us. We really had no idea of the stress and strain Grandmomma was causing him. We would ask how he was doing. He would always tell us he was OK and that he had it covered. We believed him, partly because my granddaddy could do anything. I also think we believed him because it was easier. We had jobs, children, and church. We didn't have time to help and really didn't know how.

Granddaddy soon figured out that if he was going to take care of Grandmomma, he was going to have to get sleep at night. He moved her into a nursing home. He would go there every morning and have breakfast with her. He would then take her on a ride around town, they would eat lunch, nap at home, and he would take her back and eat dinner with her before tucking her into bed at night. My grandmomma had no idea what his name was or that he had given up his family for her and her daughter. She just called him a *"Good Joe"* and *"the man who takes care of me."* As many caregivers do, my granddaddy died before my grandmomma. His body just flat wore out.

Not long after my grandparent's death, my father-in-law was diagnosed with frontal temporal lobe dementia. He was too much of a handful for my mother-in–law. We were not much help. We were stilled tied up with family and jobs. We did what we could, but we were still clueless as to resources, support, or direction. After trying a series of different assisted living communities, no placement lasting very long, she moved him to a VA home in another state. I hated that decision. To be truthful, I was angry that she did it. I have since learned how devastating caregiving can be to an individual mentally and physically. I am now an advocate for placement when the time comes. I understand that placement must happen based on the caregiver—not on the decline or abilities of the one with dementia. My father-in-law died just a few months after moving into the VA home. He went from running in the July fourth Peachtree Road Race in Atlanta to death in a VA nursing home in Alabama in fifteen months.

Shortly after my father-in-law died, my mother was diagnosed with Alzheimer's. My mother never accepted the Alzheimer's diagnosis. Not recognizing they have a problem is common for people with dementia. She felt that she was fine; everyone else, especially my dad, had a problem.

It was at this point that I started looking for a way for families to get support during their loved ones' long-term illnesses. A friend of mine led me to the Home Helpers website. There were companies that did just this! In 2006 I bought a Home Helpers franchise.

Since 2006 Home Helpers of Georgia and Alabama has helped hundreds of families. Families who learned they were not alone. Families who found support and education. Through Home Helpers, we provide in-home care for families and community workshops. We have won many awards for being the best at what we do including the Franchise of the Year award, the President's Award, and Home Care Plus certified provider and employer!

In 2013 my husband joined me in the business and in 2014 our son joined us. We operated as a family business with over a hundred well-trained, compassionate caregivers. In 2018, I handed the leadership of Home Helpers to my son so I could pursue my passion. Solutions by Beth was born out of a need for better education and understanding of the individual and family living with dementia. Solutions by Beth provides training for family members and professionals. We also provide plans for living to ensure families and individuals have a plan in place before a crisis occurs.

In the beginning, my goal was to give families support. I wanted to offer an alternative to placement for their loved ones. This book is in accordance with that goal. My hope in every conversation, talk, workshop, and now this book, is that the family living with dementia is more prepared than then they were before.

Why You Didn't See It Coming

There's always
something coming.
Good or bad. It's gonna
force you to grow.

www.Livelifehappy.com

I remember one of my boy's kindergarten teachers telling a group of us new parents of school-age children, "*If you believe half of what your children tell you about me, I will believe only half of what they tell me about you.*" As I have aged, I have found so much wisdom in that statement. It is not that people intentionally lie or mislead you. They don't tell you the truth to spare your feelings, your expectations, their pride, or mutual disappointment. People don't always give you a realistic view of their life.

This is why you didn't see it coming. Your parent may not be telling you everything about their own, or their spouse's, health. Especially if you do not live close enough to see it for yourself. And even if you are close, one spouse can "cover" for the other spouse and help hide what is really going on with their health.

I recently had a family contact me. It was a sister and brother who were concerned about their sister. The sister's husband had recently died. And while they knew that their sister had some memory loss, until the death of her husband, neither of the siblings had any idea the extent of her mental deficiencies. The recently widowed sister could not cook, remember to bathe, dress appropriately, drive, pay bills, or even tell you if she eaten or not. The family was in shock. How, and even more concerning, why, did their brother-in-law cover this up for so long? He wasn't trying to deceive anyone. His intent was not to lie. He did it out of love for his wife. So often, spouses cover for one another. It is due to a combination of denial, from both, and from wanting their loved one to always be seen in the best light to those around them.

In the early stages of my mom's dementia, whenever I would call her on the phone, she would always tell me she was ironing. My mom was a devoted military wife and the epitome of the 1950s house wife. In addition to a spotless house, she ironed everything. She even ironed my daddy's boxer shorts and t-shirts! So, my mom telling me that she was ironing was easy to believe. Until I would stop by the house and see the laundry stacked up on the bed in the spare bedroom. In her early stages, mom understood and could remember how to wash and dry clothes, but in whatever way her brain began to misfunction, what to do after the clothes came out of the dryer was no longer understood. Mom wasn't intentionally lying to me. She knew what her answer should have been. She knew what she should have been doing. She just answered the same as she had in the past.

Recognizing behavior change and not accepting the given excuses for the behavior change can open the eyes of many family members as to what is going on in the lives of their parents or older loved ones. My mom was a great cook. And her mom was a great cook. We had meals at dinner. Not one-dish casseroles, not fast food, but meals. Meat, vegetables, and dessert. Always dessert. That is how she cooked. Until she didn't. Her excuses? *There wasn't any need in cooking a big meal just for the two of them. It was easier just to go out and eat. "Microwave frozen meals are good and quick, and your daddy likes them."* And when it came to cooking for the extended family, something she loved doing in the past: *"There is just more room in the restaurant for everyone. And everyone can get what they want to eat there."* All these made sense and they could be true, for some people, but not my mom. Mom showed her love by cooking. Like her mother did. Like I do now for my family. Mom didn't stop cooking for any of the reasons she listed. She stopped cooking because she could no longer figure out how to do it all. The planning to buy the right ingredients. The order the ingredients were added. How to turn on the oven or for how long. Momma could no longer figure that out.

Men do the same thing. You often see it in their hobbies. They may have spent years in their shed out back, building stuff, fixing stuff, tinkering. But they are now spending less and less time in their shed. When they do spend time there, projects that used to turn out in days don't get completed.

There are perfectly logically reasons for the change: *"Your mom doesn't like me spending so much time out there. I just don't have time for it any more. Anything I want, I just buy it. I loaned my drill, saw, sander, out and haven't gotten it back."* The reasons make sense.

Even if you know your loved one has a memory or health issue, sometimes it is easier to believe what their spouse tells you about how they are doing day to day. Earlier I talked about how my granddaddy took care of my grandmomma until the day he died. Prior to his death I would talk to him on the phone, most of the time when he called me. I knew Grandmomma had dementia. I knew Granddaddy was taking care of her. I knew it had to be tough. But whenever I asked him about it, he always said he was good. When I asked if he needed help, or needed anything, he would say no, he had this. And I believed him. Looking back on it, I know I believed him because that was the easiest thing to do. First of all, Granddaddy could handle anything. He was a big, tough as nails, retired army sergeant … with a heart as big as his presence. He could do anything! And what could I do to help? I had a full-time job. Kids that had school and extracurricular activities that took up lots of time. We were very active in our church, which was a very active church. We lived over an hour away. We had to block out a full day just to schedule a trip. And Granddaddy "had it covered." I didn't even know what we could do to help. We didn't live close enough to help every day. What could I really do? I now know the answer. A lot. There was a lot that I could have done. And there is something you can do, whether you live across town or a hundred miles away.

If you ask your loved one if they are experiencing some memory issues, your loved one is not going to tell you the truth. Chances are, their spouse is not going to tell you the truth. By the time a person or spouse admits to you that they may be experiencing "a little dementia" or are "beginning to have some problems with short-term memory," the memory boat has sailed far into open seas.

You may not have seen it coming, but it's here now. Avoiding it will not help. Wishing it will go away will not help. Delaying choices that have to be made will not make them easier to make. When dealing with dementia, delaying a decision just makes taking action harder.

If you have a loved one with dementia, you now have one of two roles. You are either going to be the primary caregiver or you will be a support to the primary caregiver.

If you are not the primary caregiver you need to understand this: No matter what the primary caregiver is telling you, they do not have it under control. They need your help. They may not know it yet, but they will not survive this journey if they try to do it on their own.

If you are the primary caregiver, remember what you just read. You cannot do this alone. You will need help. And you will not survive if you try to do it on your own.

The Basics

If you have been on this journey for a while, this chapter may seem remedial to you. To make sure we are all on the same page I feel it necessary to include it.

One question I am asked at every talk I give, is this: *"What is the difference between Alzheimer's and dementia?"*

Dementia is a chronic, persistent disorder of the mental processes caused by brain disease or injury. Dementia is a loss of brain function. Think of it as brain failure. Dementia is a symptom. Once someone exhibits a symptom, it is important to find out what is causing the symptom. Alzheimer's is one of the brain diseases that can cause dementia. There are many others.

Think of it this way. If you go to the doctor with a runny nose, the doctor doesn't know why your nose is runny. He just sees the symptom, the runny nose. To treat you, he must find out what the illness or disease is that is causing it. Is it a cold, an allergy, an injury, or something else?

In this example, dementia is the equivalent of the runny nose. Dementia is the symptom.

Once it has been determined that someone has dementia, it is imperative to find out what is causing it. It may or may not be Alzheimer's. Too often the Alzheimer's label is given without adequate testing. There is no cure for Alzheimer's, but many forms of dementia can be treated. Dementia caused by depression, medication interactions, or even Lyme disease can be treated. With treatment the effects will diminish or go away completely. One major cause of a treatable dementia is a urinary tract infection. That's right, a simple UTI. A UTI that you can go to the drug store and buy a ten-dollar kit to detect. A UTI that most often can be treated with one round of antibiotics. A treatable, curable UTI, that if not treated, can become devastating long-lasting dementia.

If a person presents in the emergency room with Alzheimer's and hallucinations, they may be given an antipsychotic medication that will help calm them down. If this person really has Lewy body and not Alzheimer's and are given this same drug they may experience severe neuroleptic sensitivity, which could be fatal.

While there are causes of dementia that cannot be cured, what if your loved one's dementia is one of the dozen or so diseases that can be treated? Don't you want to know? Don't they deserve to know? Do not accept a dementia diagnosis without appropriate medical tests to determine the cause.

Is This My Fate Also?

Due to circumstances
beyond my control, I am
master of my fate and
captain of my soul.

Ashleigh Brilliant

When I was growing up people were so afraid of cancer they couldn't even say it. They would refer to it as the "c-word." Being diagnosed with the c-word almost surely meant death. But today, with the advances in research, medication, and treatment, cancer does not have to be a death sentence. People not only live, but can thrive, after a cancer diagnosis. Today people are afraid of the "a-word."

Especially if you have a relative with Alzheimer's. The question *am I next?* is bound to cross your mind. We see it over and over. It seems to run in families. We often see grandmothers, daughters, and granddaughters, all with the disease. We see extended family members, aunts, uncles, cousins, with the disease. Yet, the experts tell us that the only genetic link found in Alzheimer's is in those with early-onset Alzheimer's disease, which affects people younger than sixty-five years of age.

Scientists have found several rare genes that directly cause Alzheimer's. There are two types of genes that can play a role in determining if a person will develop Alzheimer's. They are risk genes and determination genes. Risk genes increase the likelihood of developing a disease but does not mean you will get it. Determination genes directly cause a disease. Determination genes guarantee that anyone who inherits the gene will develop the disease or disorder. True familial Alzheimer's disease only accounts for 1 percent of those diagnosed worldwide.

Most experts believe that Alzheimer's comes from a combination of complex interactions. Age, family history, and heredity are all risk factors that contribute to Alzheimer's. These are risk factors you cannot change. There are also lifestyle risk factors that you can do something about. There is a strong link between Alzheimer's and head trauma. So, opt for that bicycle helmet. High blood pressure, heart disease, stroke, diabetes, and high cholesterol are all factors that can contribute to your quantitative risk.

What can you do to help reduce your risk of Alzheimer's? Stay within the weight guidelines for your age and height. Avoid tobacco and excess alcohol. Stay socially connected. Exercise your mind and body. A very healthy and mentally sharp 102-year-old man once told me that he had walked thirty minutes a day every day of his life for the last 80 years. That is good enough results for me to give it a try.

Since we know that there are genes that could tell us if we are susceptible to the disease, shouldn't we all get tested? That is a decision each of you must make for yourself.

Testing may tell you if you are at risk, but remember, having the gene is not a perfect predictor of who will get the disease and who will not.

Let's say on Monday you forget where you put your car keys. You look and look and finally find them on top of the fireplace. You wonder why you put them there. You think to yourself, "*that it was a weird place to put them*" and then go on with your day. Then on Tuesday you get the results back from your blood work and you find out that you do have one of the before mentioned genes. Now losing your keys has an entirely new meaning. *"Is it starting? Did I put them there because my brain is beginning to fail? This must be the beginning."* After a positive test, every single normal forgetful thought is going to make you believe you are exhibiting symptoms of dementia. Testing for diseases you can do something about I fully understand. But Alzheimer's can't be prevented or treated. Do you really want to put yourself through the stress of thinking every time you lose your keys or forget something the disease is present and progressing?

I once had a client—a very intelligent, once active man. His family told me that he played golf almost every day. Dressed for dinner every night. Played cards and was the life of every party. Until, because of showing some symptoms, he went to his doctor and was diagnosed in the early stages of Alzheimer's. His wife told me that day her husband came home, sat in his recliner, and never participated in another activity. He felt his life was over. He went into a deep depression and isolated himself from others. He threw away two, maybe three years or more of life that he could have enjoyed, but didn't because of the diagnosis. I can very clearly see how the same thing could happen to someone if they found out that they did indeed carry a gene that might cause Alzheimer's.

All people are different. If you feel like knowing will have a positive impact on your future and help you and your family be better prepared, you may want to investigate testing. But think it through. I was given the opportunity to be tested, and knowing me, and my propensity for always thinking the worse, I chose not to be tested.

But what if you are still worried? You are forgetting more things and just don't feel as sharp as you used to be. How do you know if what you are experiencing is just aging or something more? Here is the difference. If you forget where you put your keys, even often, but can backtrack a little and soon find them, it probably isn't dementia. Contrast that to holding your car keys in your hand and not having a clue what they are or what you are supposed to do with them. The latter scenario is cause to be concerned. If you tell a joke and your friend tells you that you told them that joke a week ago, there is probably no need to worry. I have a favorite joke and I tell it every chance I get. I sometimes forget who I have told it to and wouldn't want to leave anyone out. But if you tell the same joke in the same conversation, to the same person, there may be a need to be concerned. If you can't remember what you had for lunch yesterday, join the crowd. That is just part of getting older. But if you can't remember *if* you ate breakfast, or lunch, or dinner, there may be a reason to be concerned.

As we age, we all are going to experience "senior moments." But if you have experienced any of the reasons of concern I've listed, make an appointment with your doctor.

First Steps

The first step is you have to say that you can.

Will Smith

No matter where you are on this journey of learning how to live while caring for someone with dementia, I want you to stop right now. Take a deep breath and make sure that you follow these next 8 steps. It is never too late nor too early to take them. The earlier the better, so don't put them off. These are the most important next steps you can take.

If you are the primary caregiver, you need to pull up every bit of courage and patience you can gather. Tell yourself YOU CAN DO THIS! You may have doubts. You may not know how. I'm telling you if you are realistic about your abilities, and more importantly, your limitations, you will survive this journey. It will be a journey of rewards, laughs, personal growth, and yes, sadness, but you can do this! Go ahead, say it out loud. *"I can do this!"* When you doubt it, feel overwhelmed, or feel like you can't do this another day, yell it at your loudest.

If you are not the primary caregiver I need you to understand this: The primary caregiver cannot do this on their own. No matter what they say. They will need help. Do not require more of them than you are willing to do yourself. While your help is needed in caring for the one with dementia, your first job is to care for the primary caregiver. There needs be someone one watching out for the welfare of the primary caregiver. Are they getting the sleep, medical attention, personal interaction, and support they need? Don't ever forget that all too often the primary caregiver dies before the person they are caring for—like my granddaddy, they just plain wear themselves out.

Next, learn everything you can about the diagnosis of your loved one. Every member of the family, extended family, and close friends that will play a significant role in the caregiver's and/or loved one's life should do the same. Read, Google, and go to workshops.

Third, call a mandatory family conference. This can be in person, by phone, or on FaceTime. It can be blood family and friends that are like family. The purpose of the meeting is to get everyone on the same page. Everyone needs to understand that you need their help. This is not a time for excuses about why someone cannot help. It is not the time for all the decisions about the future to be made. This is a time for, as Joe Friday would say, *"Just the facts."* Begin by explaining the dementia diagnosis. Be firm on the point that you cannot do this alone. To survive you will need help. This conversation will call for brutal honesty on your part. Many times, parents of adult children do not want their children to know their private financial situation. Good or bad. Finances are often the most difficult subject in extended family relationships. You have got to be honest here. I cannot tell you how many conversations I have been a part of where the adult children thought that their parents were financially sound, only to find that their parents' home had two mortgages and there was no savings. Caring for someone with dementia is not cheap. If everyone is going to be on the same page they need to fully understand what it is going to take to make this journey. All the cards, especially the financial cards, must be on the table.

If you need help with this conversation, there are people that can help you. Strong family friends or clergy can help lead this conversation. Geriatric care managers can also help. You can contact your local Area Agency on Aging or the Alzheimer's Association for help in your area.

Fourth, run, do not walk, to your nearest elder law attorney, financial advisor, banker, and/or veterans' care specialist. You need to know what financial resources are available to help with care. What name changes on property, bonds, etc., need to happen. Make sure all the legal paperwork, wills, trusts, and power of attorney papers are in order. If your loved one is a veteran or the spouse of a veteran, you need to know what assistance is available to help them. All too often, this step is put on the back burner. Many times, when you put something on the back burner, you forget about it. Do not delay this step.

Fifth, commit to not doing this alone. I hear folks say, *"I'll do this as long as I can."* That's like saying, *"I'm going to start cutting my arm, and when there isn't any more to cut, I'll ask someone else to take the knife."* By that time you have cut your arm off or at the very least done irreversible damage. If you do not remember anything else, remember this: caring for someone does not mean that you provide 100 percent of the care. The best care you can give your loved one may not be the care you provide. You may say, *"But my mom/ wife/husband means the world to me. I signed up for this."* How many super heroes saved the world all on their own? You must let someone else help.

Sixth, do not isolate. When you begin to care for someone, you may tend to stay home more. You are exhausted. It may be difficult to get your loved one out of the house by yourself. So, you stay home. Isolation is one of the most damaging effects caregiving has on the caregiver. It is self-sustaining, not selfish, to go to church, go out with friends, and find a support group. There are even support groups on Facebook. Find a group of people that you can help support and who can help support you.

Seventh, consider that your loved one may not be the only one that needs to be medicated. I may have just stepped on some toes there. Caregiving is stressful. One doctor said that 97 percent of all illnesses can be traced back to stress. You must survive this, for yourself and for your loved one. Go to your doctor. Get a checkup. Consider something to help you with anxiety, stress, and depression. If you needed insulin for your body to perform at its best, you would take it. So, why wouldn't you get help for the chemicals in your brain that are going haywire from the stress and exhaustion you are experiencing? Medication is not a sign of weakness. It is a show of strength that you are committed to getting through this. That you plan on being the best you can be for you and your loved one.

Last, but not least: laugh, dance, and sing! It has been proven all three of these improve your mood and help the chemicals in your brain maintain balance. Caregiving is hard but at times you can find laughter. Journaling may help. When you go back and read over the events of days past, you may find humor where you had missed it before. When there is no laughter, there is always song. Watch funny movies, sing in the shower, dance in the kitchen. Find a reason to smile.

Getting Your A-Team Together

I can do things you
cannot, you can do
things I cannot; together
we can do great things.

Mother Theresa

Most people have heard the African Proverb, "It takes a village to raise a child." The complete intended translation is, "It takes an entire community of different people interacting with children in order for children to experience and grow in a safe environment."

The same can and must be applied when caring for someone with dementia. "It takes an entire community of different people with different abilities and skills giving time to support the family living with dementia in order for both the care recipient and the caregiver to live life to their fullest abilities in a safe environment."

You are going to need a village to help you get through this: your A-team. Below is who you will need on your team.

The Planner

This person must work closely with the caregiver. The role of the planner can be filled by two people who work together. More than two people will almost never work. The planner should be a good communicator and not mind asking people to complete tasks. This person will be the one that helps place the other team members. They will need to be forward thinking and work toward always thinking about what's next. The planner may or may not live locally. Depending on the type of support you have available, this could be a very good first paid-for-hire. A geriatric care manager is the type of person who could fill this role.

The Scheduler

This is most often just one person but can be two. This person needs to be well organized. They may or may not live locally. This position is easily shared with the planner position.

The Doers

These are the boots-on-the-ground folks. It is important that each knows their task and when their task needs to be completed. You will need many of these folks on your team. As the disease progresses, you may need more skilled doers, which may require paid-for services.

The Encourager

This person is the one that always thanks everyone for doing their part. They make sure everyone remains positive and fulfilled in their individual tasks. They will make phone calls and send cards, texts, or e-mails. This person may or may not live locally.

The Financier

Not every team will have one. Some teams will have more than one. This is the team member that does not feel they have time nor talent to give but are happy to help provide financial support for whatever services are needed.

You may be thinking, *"Wait. I don't have a team that big."* These are guidelines to help you and your A-team members understand how roles can be assigned. Many times, these roles are held by one or two people. The important thing is that the roles are not filled by the primary caregiver.

Remember that your team is not in place to do the things the primary caregiver cannot do. The team is in place to do the things the caregiver doesn't *have* to do. Now if you are a natural planner and the one usually in control of day-to-day activities, it is going to be hard for you to let go. I am not saying that your team member is going to do everything the way you would do it. They may not do it as well as you could. What they will do is get it done. This will allow you time to do all the things that no one else but you can do.

Here is a list of tasks that others could do for you:
Grocery shopping
Meal prep
Laundry
Housekeeping
Yard work
Home maintenance

Driving your loved one to appointments, such as hairdresser, nail salon, etc.
Taking pets to the vet/groomer
Supervising your loved one
Scheduling bill payments

There are more. Think through your day, your week, your month, with the question, *"Is this something only I can do or can someone else do it?"* You will be able to add to this list. That being said, if something brings you joy or relaxes you, don't give it away. For example, many people find yard work cathartic. I happen to love cooking. It makes me happy. Tasks that refuel you, you will want to keep. As for the others, make a plan and give them away.

Once you have made a list of what someone other than you can do, look at the people on your A-team. Your goal is for your priority to be taking care of yourself and taking care of your loved one—in that order. You may be early enough in your journey and have an administrative, delegative type personality to get this team together. If not, it is best that the first person you identify on your team be the planner.

On the next page is a worksheet to help you build your team.

List potential team members. Not everyone you list will be on your A-team.

Beside their name put the role you think might suit them best. (P for planner, S for scheduler, D for doer, E for encourager, F for financier). You will not share this with your team members. This is to help you see how your team might fit together.

Make a list of tasks/chores that do not require you doing them.

____

____

____

____

____

____

____

____

____

____

____

____

____

____

With list in hand, approach the person you are the most comfortable with and feel most supported by. Ask them for their thoughts on the list. Add any names or tasks that they feel are missing.

Once this has been done, share the list with your team. Do not share what role you think they should fill. Ask *them* where they think they would be a good fit. You may find hidden gems in your team.

Your A-Team
The Planner:

____

____

The Scheduler:

____

____

The Doers:

____

____

____

____

____

____

____

The Encourager:

____

____

The Financier:

____

____

Your team may change. People on your team may come and go depending on their abilities and availability. Your team may be a mixture of family, friends, and paid professionals. It may also include memory care communities, nursing homes, and hospice as the disease progresses.

Out-of-Town Team Members and Paid-for Help

As I have mentioned before, team members do not have to live in your same area. Team members, or tasks, may have to be paid-for help. Here are a few examples of how to utilize a team made up of members close, far away, and paid.

Grocery Shopping: In today's world getting groceries to your door is easy. Grocery stores and discount stores have programs where you just send them a list of what you need and they will do the shopping for you. Someone can either pick it up from the store or you can have it delivered to your home. There are also apps where two or more people can share a shopping list. You just go to the app, list any items you need, and others on the shared site will check the list when they are in the store and pick them up for you.

Ordering groceries and arranging for delivery is a great job for an out-of-town team member to help you.

Meal Prep: There are healthy fresh and frozen prepared meal plans that can be delivered right to your door. There are plans where the ingredients are all delivered and you just put them together, usually taking less than thirty minutes to prepare.

If you have friends that cook regularly, they may often have left-overs. If you provide the containers they could easily freeze those and bring them over to you at the end of the week.

You can hire someone to come in and cook for you. This is not as expensive as you might think. They will typically come two times a week and make good, fresh, healthy meals for the week.

Eating right and eating healthy will be important for both the caregiver and the care recipient. Don't get trapped in fast-food, high-sodium, high-fat, low-nutrient meal plans. Meal prep is an easy fix. It can be managed by an out-of-town team member. It will save you time and help you maintain your health.

Laundry, Housekeeping, Yard Work, and Maintenance: There are for-hire services that can do these things, but often there are friends and family that will be happy to help.

Scheduling Appointments: There are many free apps available to schedule help with appointments. Someone goes into the calendar and lists the errand on the date and time needed. Members of your team can check the calendar and accept any of the assignments. These calendars are great for churches or civic organizations to help their members.

Supervising Your Loved One: As the disease progresses, much of your day will be spent making sure your loved one is safe. This is a task that really doesn't take any skill, isn't threatening, and doesn't have to require a lot of time. Many friends, family members, and church members will be more than happy to come and sit a while. During their visit you can get out or just take a nap. It is important that these times are scheduled to ensure you get the most benefit from them. These times could even be put on the calendar mentioned above.

Planning, scheduling, and assigning takes time. Let me encourage you, and your team, to think out of the box when assigning tasks. The time it gives back to the caregiver and stress it removes from the caregiver is unmeasurable.

Excuses. Excuses. Excuses.

Success is what
comes after you stop
making excuses.

Luis Galarza

I am a master excuse maker. I think it comes naturally to some of us.

Some of the best excuse-driven folks I know, second only to the student with homework due, are caregivers. Long-term caregivers often give excuses that allow them to avoid getting help. They use excuses to justify the unrealistic goal of handling the care of their loved one all by themselves. Therefore, not needing to build a team.

I want to take a minute to look at some of these excuses you may have heard others use, and if you are already in the caregiver role, you may have used a few yourself.

Excuse number one: *"I don't need a break."* Even God took a break on the seventh day! All of us need a break to recharge or rest. Caregivers are no different. Forty to seventy percent of long-term caregivers die before the person they are taking care of dies. This gap in the statistic is due to the age and health of the caregiver. Very often the caregiver is not in good health. They are just in better health than the person receiving care. Taking better care of yourself, getting rest, eating healthy meals, and taking care of your own needs helps you take better care of your loved one. Even just an hour away from the responsibility of caregiving can mean a world of difference.

I will tell you a secret. Not only will that break be good for you, it will be good for your loved one. They need a break from you, too! The more time you spend together, patience can begin to wear thin. Your loved one has no idea what they have done or said to cause the short-tempered response from you. Face it, after being asked the same question twenty times, even the strongest of us would have a tendency to snap. This is a marathon. The only way to sustain the love and care you feel your loved one deserves is to take good care of yourself. Taking care of yourself means taking a break.

Schedule a break on your calendar. If you are like me if it is not on my calendar it will not happen. This is the time to utilize friends, family members, home care services, and adult day programs. Your A-team. I know what you're thinking: *"I just hate to ask them."* Get over it! Most people really don't mind helping. They just don't know what to do or how to help. Getting away could be having someone over for thirty minutes while you go outside and sit in the sun. It will be OK, and you will see that your loved one can make it without you. Then you can move to longer periods of time and even get off the property. Whomever you need to get to help you, however you need to plan it, the important thing is to plan it and go!

Excuse number two: *"It will cause me more stress."* This excuse is often given when you ask a caregiver about adult day programs or bringing someone into the home. It just isn't true. I have had caregivers in my home twenty-four seven. It takes some getting used to, but it is not more stressful than trying to do everything on my own. Your loved one may not want anyone in their home. They may just want you to help them. Believe me, they will get past that. I cannot tell you how many times a family caregiver has told me that our caregiver in their loved ones' home wouldn't last an hour. But they do. Sometimes it is tough. Sometimes you have to go through a couple of different caregivers. Once the caregiver and care recipient get used to each other, it really does work. The stress this extra set of hands relieves is unbelievable!

If you choose an adult day program it may make for a hectic morning. If transportation is not offered that could be an extra hassle. Compare that to the six to eight hours of caring-free time you will get in return, the stress a day program could relieve is significant. Don't fall for the *"you're just sending me to a babysitter"* response from your loved one. Your loved one will have a blast, feel better, and have a better quality of life. One risk of aging and illness is isolation. Being with people and keeping social has proven to help reduce depression and help people live longer. Don't expect your loved one to tell you they are having a good time. They will tell you that no one talks to them, that they are bored, or that they don't do anything. I have a friend whose mom told her all these things. Unfortunately for her mom, the community had a big bulletin board that always showed pictures of past events. Her mom was always in the pictures front and center with a big smile.

Excuse number three: *"I can't afford help."* There is low-cost and even free help available. It may take some creativity and research, but it is so worth it. If your care recipient is a veteran or the spouse of a veteran, check out the Aid and Attendance benefit. Medicaid will pay for limited home care. Many adult day programs are based on ability to pay. Never underestimate the willingness of friends or other family members to give a few hours of their time to give you a break. And don't forget the financier on your team. Their funding can pay for help. Contact your local Area Agency on Aging for community programs that may offer support. Yes, care is costly. Often the personal cost of not getting help will outweigh the cost of care.

Excuse number four: *"I promised I would never put her in a home."* If you have not made this promise to your loved one, don't! If you have made this promise, don't let that promise bind you to the unrealistic goal of caring for your loved one all by yourself. If your loved one has pleaded with you not to put them "in a home," you must first understand their fears. Their opinion of a "home" is often the industrialized, sterile, dark facilities of the past. Not the beautiful, bright, lively communities of today. Second, they fear being alone. They are afraid that they will no longer see you. Help them to understand that not only will they see you, but when they do see you, you will be able to spend your time with them being their child, their spouse, their sibling, not their caregiver. Your job is to provide the best care for your loved one. The best care may not be the care you can give them.

Excuse number five: *"No one will look after her/him like I will."* I have twenty-four-hour care for my mom. I know without a doubt that they provide better care for her than I could ever give her. Her care is shared by caregivers that get breaks. When they come in for a shift, they are fresh and ready for the day, not already exhausted.

If you are a caregiver on this journey, stop the excuses and allow others to help. If you are a friend or family member to a caregiver, don't let them continue to make excuses. Help them find their success.

What You Need to Know

Be strong enough to
stand alone, smart
enough to know when
you need help, and brave
enough to ask for it.

In school, there are three basics: reading, writing, and arithmetic. These three subjects are the foundation for all your other learning. In the next pages I will lay the groundwork for a strong foundation. Remember, there is no book, no conference, no conversation that will tell you everything you need to know about living with a loved one with dementia. Read as much as you can. Learn as much as you can. Then share what you have learned with others. That is how we as families get through this journey.

Anosognosia

Your loved one will not believe that there is anything wrong with them. This is not denial. Damage to the brain caused by disease or injury can cause them to believe that there is nothing wrong with them. This is called anosognosia. Do not try to convince them; it will not help.

It is OK to Lie

I know that you have been raised to always tell the truth. The world of dementia has different rules. In the world of dementia, it is often more kind to lie. If your loved one wants to go somewhere, and it is not possible for you to take them, do not tell them "no" and begin an argument. Tell them that you will take them tomorrow. If your loved one has forgotten that their spouse has died, and they ask you where their spouse is, why tell them they are dead? This will just cause your loved one pain. Tell them that their spouse is at the store or work. In many cases it is more compassionate to not tell them the truth.

Guns

The person with dementia should never be in a home where guns are accessible. I don't care how mad you think your loved one may get at the removal of the guns. If there are guns in the home, your loved one may get to them. If your loved one gets to the guns they may use them against you, a grandchild, or themselves. It is amazing how often guns are removed from a home and the person with dementia is never aware they are missing. There are no exceptions to this no-gun rule.

Driving

If your loved one has dementia they must not drive. Removing driving privileges is hard, but for their safety and the safety of others it must be done. While you must remove their right to drive, you must not remove their right to transportation. Before you take their keys away, have a plan for how they will get where they need and want to go.

Triggers

Your loved one will have certain "triggers." If you can figure out what they are, it will make life easier for both of you. I know this may sound odd, but believe me, items can trigger behaviors. Keys can be a trigger that they need to drive. Just as a car in the driveway may be a trigger. Remove the keys or the car from sight, and the mental cue that they are supposed to or want to drive is gone. My father-in-law drove much longer than we should have allowed him. He got in his truck every day and drove somewhere. One day we moved his truck to the back of the property, out of his sight. From that day, he didn't remember that he was supposed to drive.

Pictures of family members even pictures of your loved one around the house, could trigger anxiety. They may no longer recognize the people in the pictures that are surrounding them. This could trigger confusion and anxiety.

Clutter in a home can be a trigger, especially if the person with dementia was always very neat. You may not understand what is causing their anxiety. It could be something as simple as the newspaper laying on the floor.

When you notice a behavior, especially a repetitive behavior, look for the trigger that may be causing it.

Bathroom Habits

If your loved one with dementia is over the age of sixty, they may go to the bathroom in a garbage can. This is very common. Many of us of a certain age can remember back to the day of outhouses. If you had an outhouse, you didn't necessarily go out to use the bathroom at night. You would use a jar, or a bucket, an item that might look a lot like a garbage can today. Remove the garbage can, remove the trigger and the problem.

They Are Going to Use Foul Language

There are a couple of reasons this happens. One reason is because dementia affects different parts of the brain at different times. When damage occurs to the frontal lobe, the filter part of our brain will no longer work correctly. The part of their brain that tells them what to say or what not to say is gone. Therefore, whatever comes to mind comes out of the mouth.

The second reason your loved one will cuss is because our brains process language on the right side of the brain. The personality-connected emotion processing is done on the left side of your brain. Processing language is a higher brain function. Processing emotion is a lower instinctual brain function. This means if the dementia reaches the right, higher functioning side of the brain first, cuss words are apt to fly. This, like all other dementia behaviors, cannot be controlled. Chastising your loved one, correcting them, or trying to shame them for their language is not constructive. It is the disease, not your loved one.

Valuables

Once your loved one has been diagnosed with dementia, remove anything of value from their surroundings. People with dementia do not know the value of items. They give away items, hide items, and throw items away. Many times, things of value have been lost because the person with dementia has been allowed to continue to have access to them. Wedding rings or any jewelry of value should be replaced with cheap "dime store" jewelry. Money, collections, and any other items of value should be removed. This step needs to be taken early.

Your loved one needs to have limited ability to access funds from their bank account. All credit cards should be closed. They should not be allowed to carry large sums of cash. If they are used to carrying cash, give them ten one-dollar bills.

Security

If your loved one lives alone, place a camera at all exterior doors. You need to know who is coming to their door and you need to know if your loved one leaves.

If you move your loved one into a nursing home, a memory care community, or if you bring help into the home, place a hidden camera to monitor how people interact with them. Most communities will have policies against hidden surveillance. If they find out you have a hidden camera, they will most likely give you notice that your loved one will have to move. I recommend you place the camera anyway.

Visual Field and Clarity

Your loved one's visual field will shrink. Hold your hands up to your eyes as if you are using them as binoculars. Notice how your peripheral vision is restricted? If you are sitting at a table, you will not be able to see what is on the table closest to you. If you look straight ahead at a person standing in front of you, you will only see their torso, not their face. If someone was to comes up beside you and put their hand on your shoulder, you would not see them coming and could be startled.

When you are approaching your loved one, be sure that you approach them from the front and in a straight shot of their visual range. This may mean that you will need to bend down a little and not stand too close to them.

When serving them a meal be sure they can see their plate. When my father-in-law was alive he would always eat off everyone else's plate. He wouldn't touch his plate, no matter how often we reminded him it was in front of him. The problem we didn't recognize was that he couldn't see his plate. He ate off the plates he could see.

Just as their visual field is shrinking, their brightness and clarity is reducing. This means that colors will lose their contrast. Everything will appear dull. Objects that could be seen before will now blend into the background. For example: white mashed potatoes on a white plate; a brown ottoman on a brown carpeted floor; a pale-yellow towel next to a similarly colored wall.

Brightly colored plates will make foods easier to recognize. Bright placemats will help define the area between the plate and the table. A bright seat cushion will help distinguish the seat from the floor. Bright colors will help their brain better react to depth, as their depth perception also becomes an issue.

Look at your loved one's living environment. Create contrast with bright colors.

Sundowning

Sundowning occurs in the late afternoon and early evenings. It is a time when your loved one will become agitated and anxious. It happens due to a combination of events. Think about what occurs in early afternoon/late evening. Energy wise, you hit a wall. If you work, you are beginning the transition from finishing work to starting your travel home. You may have to fight traffic. Your kids are getting home from school, you have after school activities and at-home work. You have dinner to cook, or pick up, yard work to do, and laundry. Then there are baths and the nightly bedtime battles. For the average adult this late afternoon/ early evening time is a busy time. It is go, go, go. Take that average adult and give them dementia. Their body tells them it is go, go, go time, but there is nowhere to go, go, go. They don't know what they are supposed to be doing. They just have this urge that they are supposed to be doing something. They don't know what it is, you don't know what it is, and anger and frustration occur.

While there is medication that can help with the symptoms of sundowning, you may want to try a few other things. First, try not to have overly exhausting days. This goes for both of you. When tired, we all can become more quick tempered and easily agitated. Throw in a little dementia, and you can both really get on each other's last nerve. If you have had an exhausting day, you really need to call for back-up and get help with your loved one. You being tired can have a strong negative effect on their sundowning. Bringing in someone fresh to be with them during this time could make a big change for both of you.

When planning your days, accept that it will take twice as long to do anything with a person with dementia. Rushing is not going to help. Limit your errands. Don't try to do multiple things in one day. Set aside extra time for the unexpected. There may be times during the day that your loved one feels better and responds better. You should schedule all your outings during those times. If your loved one is not a morning person, running errands in the morning may cause them to be tired all day and can set the stage for a rough sundowning period.

Have activities available for this time. A basket full of towels and washcloths to fold will give them something meaningful to do. A tool box with nails, nuts, and bolts that need organizing will do the same. My mom could spend hours, yes hours, reading and sorting mail. A small stack, over and over. When their body is telling them that they need to be doing something, give them something to do.

Turn on the lights. As the sun goes down shadows can appear in the home. These shadows can cause confusion and fear. They may be perceived to be something that will cause your loved one harm.

If your loved one tells you that they need to "pick the kids up from school," just remind them that the kids had practice after school today, went home with a friend today to work on a school project, or any other reasonable excuse for why they do not have to go get the kids. Do not tell them that they do not have kids to pick up. In their mind they do. You telling them they don't will only agitate them more. Remember from earlier, it is often more compassionate to not tell the whole truth.

Delusions and Paranoia

As your loved one's dementia progresses, it will be harder and harder for them to remember the current. This creates confusion as to what is happening around them. Your loved one will try to make sense of it and this will often lead to being delusional and paranoid. A delusion is believing something that is not true. Paranoia is often the results of the delusion.

Your loved one with dementia may remember distinctly and correctly that they have fifty dollars in their wallet. The problem is that memory was a memory from five years ago. They think it is a memory from today. So, if their fifty dollars is missing the only logical explanation for them is that someone took it.

If your loved one accuses you of taking something, assure them that you would not take it. Then help them look for it. You can offer to call people that may have seen "it." You can even offer to call the authorities about the missing item.

The best way to handle their delusions and paranoia is to help them find resolution. Help them hunt for the ring, the wallet, the money, for as long as it takes. As with most dementia behaviors, it is better to join in than to fight it.

Are They Left Handed or Right Handed?

As the disease progresses, your loved one will need to be bathed or fed. It will feel more natural to your loved one and easier to accept if the act is approached from your loved ones dominate hand side. If they are right handed, feed them from the right. Bathe them from the left if they are left handed.

If They Want to Go, Go

Do not try to prevent your loved one from leaving a room or the residence. If your loved one is determined to leave, and you try to stop them, one of you is likely to get hurt. It is fine to try to redirect them once or twice. If they are insistent on leaving, and if their agitation rises, it is best just to let them go. If you are not prepared for it, this can be disastrous.

Plan for when your loved one insists on leaving. Prior to this behavior contact neighbors near and in the neighborhood. Let them know that your loved one is at risk for wanting to leave. Ask if you can call them and have them intercept your loved one if this happens. Advise them not to chase after your loved one, but to greet them with a smile. Have them ask if they can walk with them, or if they would to come in for a drink or a visit. They can even greet them with a *"Hi, I've been waiting on you."*

If you do not have people you can ask to help, you contact your local police or sheriff's office. Be sure they completely understand the situation. Advise them not to run lights or sirens. They should stop well ahead of your loved one and approach them from the front in a *"Hi, how are you doing"* manner. They should present themselves as a friend or companion. Not someone trying to stop their progression.

When your loved one leaves, go with them. Do not chase them. Offer to go with them to help them find what or who they are searching for. If you determine that you are not going to be able to get them circled back home, or if they become aggressive or panicked by your presence, contact either your neighbor or the police for help.

Eventually they will forget why they are going and you will be able to redirect them home.

This "needing to go" is a phase that almost all people with dementia will go through. It can be freezing outside or raining, and they may walk for hours. It is not fun, but as mentioned before, if you can join the behavior and not fight it, the end result will be best for both of you.

You Have to Pick Your Battles

In the scheme of things, some things just are not so important any more. Keep that in mind. I remember answering the phone when I was running my home care agency and hearing a woman yelling at me about how our caregiver had allowed her mother-in-law to go out of her apartment in black pants and brown socks. The daughter-in-law was livid. I'm sorry, but in a world where just getting your loved one dressed is a win, their socks not matching their pants is not a big deal. If clothes matching is important to you, get them a new wardrobe of all black or khaki pants and shirts that will match. Buy one color of socks that matches the color of the pants. Make it easy.

If your loved one wants to wear their bra on the outside of their shirt and you aren't planning on going anywhere that day, why does it matter? If they want to wear the same outfit three days in a row, and it is not soiled, is it worth the fight? Probably not. Now on the fourth day, you do have my permission to spill cold coffee, milk, or soda on them. Accidentally, of course. They will change on their own.

The Cost of Care

Paid for services range in costs depending on where you live and the type of services your loved one will need. As a rule of thumb, non-medical in-home care, provided by a licensed agency will average $18 to $25 an hour. You can find a private caregiver to provide these services. The average paid-for unlicensed private caregiver will range from $8 to $15 an hour. If you do hire a private caregiver, do not do so without references and a background check. By law the private caregiver must be considered an employee with all the appropriate taxes withheld and paid. They are not a 1099 contractor for several reasons; one being they are not in control of their schedule. They are working for you. Do not skirt labor rules. It can come back to bite you and cause you stress and money.

Medicare does not pay for in-home, non-medical care. Medicaid will pay for a limited amount of non-medical in-home care. Medicaid is needs based.

The cost of assisted living and memory care varies greatly. Most are private pay. The cost for these communities range from $4000 a month $8000, and more, a month.

Medicaid, not Medicare, pays for long-term nursing home stay. Medicaid is based on the financial need of the person. At present, for a person to qualify for nursing home care, they can make up to 300 percent of the SSI income limit. (300 percent of the SSI limit, $750, is $2,250 per month.)

Aide and Attendance is a VA benefit for veterans and their spouses. This is a need-based benefit and requires that the veteran served during war-time and was honorably discharged.

The Death Certificate Matters

Alzheimer's dementia is the leading cause of death in England and Wales. It has more than doubled since 2010. In the US Alzheimer's is the sixth leading cause of death overall and the fifth leading cause of death in those over sixty-five years of age. Why the difference? Are Alzheimer's and other forms of dementia more rampant in England and Wales than here in the US?

Medical or health complications from illness are caused or exacerbated by Alzheimer's disease and other dementias. Alzheimer's disease, as well as other dementias, cause brain failure. With brain failure comes organ failure (example: heart and lungs), digestive failure, immune system failure, and failure of other bodily functions. Most often the cause of death of someone with dementia is a secondary infection (usually pneumonia), organ failure, heart attack, dehydration and malnutrition, injuries or fractures, stroke, kidney failure, or sepsis (like a urinary tract infection).

When death occurs, the medical examiner fills out the death certificate and writes the cause of death as the last malady that ended the person's life. Even if dementia was the dominate factor in the decline of the individual, it may not appear on the death certificate. It is imperative that we ensure the specific dementia diagnosis is listed on our loved one's death certificate. Statistics come from the death certificates. More importantly, funding comes from the statistics. A number-one cause of death is going to get more attention, more funding, and more research than a sixth-leading cause of death. If dementia was listed on death certificates in every incident where it was the origin of the eventual cause of death, I truly feel that we would find that the number-one cause of death in the US would be a form of dementia. We might even find that Lewy body dementia would beat out Alzheimer's as number one.

When your loved one dies, tell the medical examiner (or hospice nurse) that you want their specific type of dementia listed on the death certificate. The immediate cause of death will be listed. Dementia must also get placed on the certificate.

Being a Medical Advocate

Unless someone like you
cares a whole awful lot,
nothing is going to get
better. It's not.

Dr. Seuss, The Lorax

In the early stages of dementia, doctor visits and the consumption of medication may not be an issue. As your loved one declines, securing medical attention and getting them to properly take their medication will become more difficult. There may come a time when you must weigh the benefits of the medication, medical tests, and procedures. Compared to the stress, strain, and quality of life each is working to prolong, is it worth it.

Doctor Visits/ Testing/ Procedures

If there is any way you can avoid the doctor's office when your loved one is ill, do it. Today there are concierge medical services that will come to your home. They accept Medicare, Tricare, and most insurances. They can give IVs, diagnose many conditions, and they can do x-rays in your home. Having your loved one seen, diagnosed, and treated in the comfort of their own home is always less stressful.

If you do have to go into the doctor's office, be sure the staff understands the condition of your loved one and the need to not wait in the waiting room. The unfamiliar faces and noises in the waiting room, in addition to waiting in the exam room with the door closed for long periods of time, is a recipe for stress and anxiety. Helping the office staff understand the need for expediency in the visit may take a face-to-conversation. This conversation should take place prior to the appointment. You should ask them to flag your loved one's file so whoever is scheduling the visit will understand the parameters.

If possible, always try to take a third party with you to the doctor. If your loved one does get antsy and needs to walk out one of you can stay and wait for their turn to be seen.

If your loved one doesn't want to go to the doctor or says they don't need to go, it sometimes works for you to tell them that the doctor visit is for you.

If it is hard for you to speak freely to the doctor in front of your loved one be sure to communicate any issues or concerns outside of earshot of your loved one. This can often be done by a prior e-mail or letter written and handed to the front desk upon check-in.

Once your loved one has been diagnosed with dementia, normal, regular medical visits and testing may no longer be necessary. Mammograms, Pap smears and colonoscopies may no longer make sense. If a medical exam or test results in a need for a medical procedure you will need to decide if having the procedure is what is best for your loved one. A person with dementia cannot properly metabolize anesthesia. Whatever their mental processes are before their surgery their mental abilities after the anesthesia will be reduced and often reduced significantly. If, after surgery, physical rehabilitation is required your loved one may not have mental capacity to complete the rehabilitation. Therefore, never fully recovering physically in addition to the mental decline from the procedure. For the person with dementia, lifesaving surgeries may only prolong a life that is lived without sufficient brain function. You will have to decide if that is what is best for your loved one.

Medication

Two issues are typically presented with medications. Your loved one will refuse to take their medications, or they no longer understand how to swallow their medications. Both cases can be stress filled. If it is early in the disease process you may decide to crush their medications and hide them in another substance. Keep in mind that as the disease progresses you may want to consult their doctor and decide if all your loved one's medications are necessary.

Hospital Stays

In my perfect world every hospital will have a dementia care team. This DCT will be assigned to patients brought into the hospital with a diagnosis, or suspicion, of dementia. The DCT will work closely with the patient, their family, and the hospital staff. Every hospital will have a separate protocol for the dementia patient. I hope my one day comes soon. Until then, you as the primary caregiver must gain the knowledge and have the confidence to speak out and stand up for your loved one. This will ensure they receive the best care possible is a dementia-friendly environment.

I understand hospital protocol and the right to patient confidentiality. I understand rules. I understand the need for rules. I also understand what it is like to be scared, alone, and not understood. If there is anything I can do to minimize those feelings in a loved one, I will do whatever I need to do. I encourage you to have the confidence to do the same.

Every person that enters the patient's room should know that the person has dementia. Whether that is a sign on the door, a tag on their chart, or, my personal choice, a special color of hospital gown.

Since I mentioned hospital gown, why not start there? If the patient with dementia does not want to wear a hospital gown, if they fight to put it on, or if they keep trying to take it off, and if it is not a matter of life and death, let them wear their street clothes. If necessary for the patient to wear a hospital gown, wait until is it night and time to change into pajamas. Tell your loved one that you forgot their pajamas, but they can wear "this gown" until you bring theirs. This will often make the transition from clothing to hospital gown easier.

When someone is checked into a hospital room the room immediately fills with activity. There are multiple people asking questions, pulling and tugging on your loved one. These are all anxiety-creating activities. If possible, there should only be one hospital staff person at a time in the patient's room. Any questions that can be asked outside of the patient's room and answered by someone other than the dementia patient (i.e. name, birthdate, what brings you here today, etc.) should be done outside. I understand the need for vitals, bloodwork, and medical history but when caring for someone with dementia, a little deviation from normal hospital routine can go a long way in helping the patient react positively to their stay.

All noise-creating systems need to be turned off in your loved one's room. If there is a hospital intercom system that goes off in each room, it needs to be turned off. If there is a bed alarm that goes off loudly when the patient leaves the bed, it needs to be exchanged with a silent alarm. If there are speakers in the room that play sweet lullaby music each time a baby is born, it needs to be turned off. IV trees should be turned off so they do not beep when a medication is completed. Because excess noise is not understood, it is anxiety-building for the dementia patient and should be avoided when possible.

Hospital rooms are often cluttered. Clutter is confusing. Your loved one can easily become overwhelmed from not understanding what everything is, what they are supposed to do with it, and with just having it invade their area.

Your loved one's bed should always be placed in the lowest position, closet to floor, when they are left alone. If capable, your loved one will leave their bed. Having the bed at the lowest level will help prevent falls.

If your loved one must have an IV, you need to request a full "sleeve" on their IV arm. Your loved one will see the sleeve, not the IV. They will not be able to play or pull at the IV, reducing the risk of it being pulled out.

If you cannot have someone be with your loved one in their room twenty-four seven, there are times more vital than others. During meal time, during staff shift changes, and during the later afternoon to evening hours your loved one should not be alone.

I was amazed when I heard how many senior adults enter hospitals malnourished. I found a 2015 statistic that said it was one in six. It is not a huge jump to believe that people with dementia enter the hospital with a rate equal if not higher. What is hard to understand and somewhat counterintuitive is that these malnourished patients leave the hospital more malnourished than when they arrived. Knowing this, it also makes sense that many seniors with dementia return to the hospital within thirty to sixty days after discharge.

So how do seniors, especially seniors with dementia, leave the hospital more malnourished than when they went in? You know the drill. The dinning staff comes into the room. Shows the patient their food and puts it on their bed tray. They position the tray for eating and leave. In an hour or so they come back. If the food has not been eaten, they ask, "Were you not hungry?" The person with dementia often does not recognize the feelings of hunger or thirst. What they may still understand is when asked a question, if they smile or nod or shake their head or say no, people leave them alone Then the tray is removed. Just being in the hospital is confusing enough. The food tray does not look like how their plate at home looks. It is covered and for the person with dementia, if you can't see it, it isn't there. Once the dining staff leaves, the dementia patient may no longer recognize it as their meal. If they do recognize it as their meal, they may not understand that they have permission to eat. They may not understand how to use the utensils. And so, when it is time for the next meal the results are the same. Day after day.

Having someone with them to encourage them to eat and drink is imperative to ensure they receive the nourishment that will give them the strength needed to heal or at least to not return home in worse condition. If family and friends are not available during meal time, arrange for meals to be provided while someone is with them. You may want to consider paying an agency to provide someone to be with them. Meal time is the most vital time for your loved one to have someone with them to ensure they are getting the nutrition they need to heal.

Shift change is the next most important time for someone to have eyes on your loved one. If your loved one is an elopement risk—and sooner or later, with no warning, most people with dementia will be an elopement risk—shift change is a perfect time for them to wander off without being noticed. Needs that your loved one feels are urgent may go unaddressed, causing additional stress and anxiety and fueling the need to escape. Even if your loved one does not leave their room they can work themselves into a state of delirium.

Sundowning usually occurs in the late afternoon through the early evening hours. During sundowning your loved one will be anxious and unsure of what they need to be doing. They know they are supposed to be doing something. They will often pace uncontrollably, have bursts of anger, are more confused, and can be hard to control. In the hospital this time is often exasperated by shift changes and hospital policies. I was recently in a hospital that had "quiet time" to "promote healing" from three to five every evening. During that time, they dimmed the lights, lowered the window shades, and reduced the amount of hall traffic.

For the person sundowning, the last thing they need is a dimly lit room.

The effects off sundowning can be greatly reduced by having a person with them.

Hospice

Don't let the word scare you. Hospice does not mean you have given up on your loved one. It does not mean that your loved one is going to die soon. Hospice is a wonderful service that will provide you and your loved one support, supplies, RN home visits, personal visits, and more. All to ensure that your loved one's final phase of their journey is compassionate, comfort-filled, and supported for both of you.

What People Don't Tell You

It's like I want you
to know, but I don't
want to tell you.

Unknown

There are some topics and feelings that people do not talk about. You may have feelings that you do not understand and may even be embarrassed by. Your loved one may do things that you can't understand. The life lived in the dementia world is not always normal. No matter how alone you feel in your emotions as you go through this journey, know that you are not alone. Your emotions, their actions, are normal in this new world.

They Will Forget Who You Are

No matter how prepared you try to be when your loved one does not know who you are, the pain is beyond what you will expect. You will feel deeply hurt that they do not remember you. Sometimes, they may remember one child and not the other. They may remember their ex-husband and not their present husband. You will wonder why. You will wonder if they loved you less, if you meant less to them. Who they forget first or last doesn't have anything to do with the amount of love they had for that person. You know this day will come, and intellectually you understand it. However, when the day arrives, it will hurt beyond your expectations.

They May Fall in Love with Someone Else

If the time comes and you move your loved one into a memory care community, there is a strong possibility that they may have a romantic relationship with one of the other residents. It is hard to see your spouse of sixty years holding hands and singing to another. Looking at them the way they used to look at you. You will feel betrayed. You will feel hurt. In your head you know that it is because their brain has scrambled their years and brought them to a world where you do not exist. Where the relationship the two of you had is no longer in their memory. In your heart you will still feel the pain.

You Want It to Be Over

You will be ready for them to die. You may even want them to die. This is a long and hard journey. At the end, there may only be a shell where your loved one used to live. They have been gone for a very long time. You will be tired. You will be ready for it to be over. The only way for it to be over is for your loved one to die. You will feel guilty that this thought crossed your mind. You will hate yourself for having this thought. You may question what type of person, spouse, child, or sibling you are to feel this way. You are not alone. This is normal.

You May Fall Out of Love

You may no longer love this person. You love who they were. You will love the relationship you had with them. One day, you may not feel love toward the person that is in front of you. You need to know, that is OK. The body that is in front of you is not the person you loved in the prior years. That person is gone. This does not make you a bad person.

You Will Feel Like an Orphan

Even though they are still alive, you will feel like an orphan. People won't understand that feeling. They will say things to you like, "*You are so blessed to still have your mom.*" You haven't had your mom for a very long time. Her body may still be living but your mom has died.

No One Will Ask

People are not going to ask you how you are. They are going to ask you how your loved one with dementia is doing. If your loved one is a parent, they will ask you how your other parent is doing. Your children will ask you how their dad or mom or grandparent with dementia is feeling. They won't ask about you. It will be easy for you to believe that how you are doing doesn't matter. No one will seem to notice that you are grieving. If your loved one had died, people would understand your loss. They would talk to you about it and sympathize with your grief. When your loved one has dementia, their body is still alive. Therefore, people do not recognize your grief. They do not understand. This is why support groups are so important. You need to have people around you who understand.

Making Love

You may still make love with your spouse with dementia. You may wonder if you are taking advantage of them. You may be afraid that others may think you are taking advantage of them. This is your spouse, making love is how the two of you have celebrated your love in the past, when life was normal. If your loved one with dementia does not say no or does not appear to be afraid, it is OK if you make love to your spouse.

You may not want to make love with your spouse. You just changed their diaper ten minutes earlier. They have forgotten but you have not. You may feel sorry for them but the thought of making love is close to disgusting to you. You are human. You are going through a whirlwind of emotions and feelings that change from day to day. This is normal.

You May Have Feelings for Someone New

If you are the spouse of someone with dementia, you may find yourself in a relationship with someone else. Others may not understand. You are, after all, still married. You may feel guilty for thinking about someone other than your spouse. Wanting to love someone and wanting someone to love you is normal. Yes, you are still married. However, the person you married, the person you were in love with, no longer exists. Falling in love with someone else while your spouse with dementia is still alive has nothing to do with the amount of love you had for that person during your life together. You still have a life to live. Do not allow dementia to end your life. Everyone needs to feel love.

Strained Relationships with Siblings

You may resent your siblings who you do not feel are pulling their weight. Your siblings may resent you for not doing everything they think you should be doing. You will question their motives at times, and they will question yours. You will never completely agree on the best plan of care for your parent. Having a parent with dementia may cause strain on a good sibling relationship. For a relationship that is already strained, it may cause severe damage.

Your Feelings Will Get Hurt

Your loved one is going to say things to you that will hurt you to your core. You will try to remember that it is the disease and not them, but it will still hurt.

Final Thoughts

Always remember that
your present situation is
not your final destination.

Zig Ziglar

If you have children, you may be familiar with the feeling you get in the pit of your stomach when they have been hurt by someone. When you find that your loved one has dementia you will begin to feel that same type of pain form in your gut. As you go through this dementia journey with them, that pain will begin to feel like a hole in your soul. I wish I could tell you how to fix that hole—or better yet, prevent it from forming. I can't. I can tell you that the size of the hole is not permanent and will shrink over time.

Dementia not only takes away brain function from our loved ones, it takes away a piece of us. We are not the same after caring for a loved one with dementia. Life is more precious. We live life wondering if it's our fate as well. We worry that dementia will claim other members of our family.

The different forms of dementia are diseases that we must never stop fighting against. Learn as much as you can.

Share as much as you can. Join the fight for a cure. A cure will come.

Most of all, survive this journey. There is life after caregiving. Share your knowledge and experiences with others. We would not know today what we know if it wasn't for those who came before us. After you have finished your journey, help someone who is just beginning theirs. For that is how we get through this, helping one another. Giving advice, inspiration, and most importantly, understanding.

Made in the USA
Columbia, SC
11 September 2023

22739070R00043